WHO/HTM/TB/2006.363

Tuberculosis and air travel

Guidelines for prevention and control

SECOND EDITION

World Health Organization

WHO Library Cataloguing-in-Publication Data

Tuberculosis and air travel : guidelines for prevention and control. – 2nd ed. –

"... prepared by WHO in collaboration with the International Civil Aviation Organization, the International Air Transport Association, international experts in tuberculosis and other infectious diseases, and leading authorities in public health and travel medicine" – Acknowledgements.

"The preparation of the guidelines was coordinated by Kwon Jun Wook"– Acknowledgements.

"WHO/HTM/TB/2006.363".

1.Tuberculosis – prevention and control. 2.Tuberculosis – transmission. 3.Aircraft. 4.Travel. 5.Guidelines. I.Wook, Kwon Jun. II.World Health Organization. III.International Civil Aviation Organization. IV.International Air Transport Association.

ISBN 92 4 154698 0 (NLM classification: WF 200)
ISBN 978 92 4 154698 0

First edition, 1998
Second edition, 2006

Designed by minimum graphics
Printed in France

Contents

Preface

Air travel is now widely accessible, resulting in increasing numbers of international air travellers, with a consequent increased risk of the spread of infectious diseases carried by infected travellers. Transmission of airborne infection between people in confined spaces such as aircraft cabins is of particular concern to health officials and the public at large.

In the early 1990s, there were reports of the transmission during long flights of tuberculosis (TB) infection, including its most dangerous form, multidrug-resistant TB (MDR-TB), from contagious travellers to other passengers and crew. These episodes caused anxiety among travellers and serious concern among public health officials and airline companies. The World Health Organization (WHO) published guidelines in 1998 defining the extent of the problem and the potential risks and providing recommendations for travellers, physicians and health authorities and airline companies. The recommendations were based on the limited experience available at the time: investigations involving seven contagious TB patients and some 2600 potentially exposed air travellers.

Since attention has been drawn to the risk of TB transmission on board aircraft, other airborne diseases have caused major international public health emergencies, in some cases involving the actual or potential of transmission of infection during international flights. In addition, the emergence of MDR-TB in recent years has raised special concerns in relation to the international spread of particularly dangerous strains of *Mycobacterium tuberculosis*. It is therefore increasingly necessary to have clear and effective procedures in place to reduce the risk of transmission of infection on board and to ensure appropriate follow-up when necessary.

The revised International Health Regulations, adopted in 2005, provide a legal framework for a more effective coordinated international response to emergencies caused by outbreaks of infectious diseases. A number of provisions are relevant to the detection and control of TB during air travel, strengthening the authority of WHO and of national public health authorities in this domain.

Because of these important developments since the original guidelines were issued in 1998, WHO has prepared this revised version to take account of current public health risks that may arise during air travel and new approaches to international collaboration in dealing with them. The guidelines were developed with the collaboration of international experts in air travel medicine and other authorities. Implementing the recommendations will help to reduce the spread of dangerous pathogens across the globe and decrease the risk of infection among individual travellers.

Mario Raviglione
Director
Stop TB Department
World Health Organization

Acknowledgements

This second edition of *Tuberculosis and air travel: guidelines for prevention and control* was prepared by WHO in collaboration with the International Civil Aviation Organization, the International Air Transport Association, international experts in tuberculosis and other infectious diseases, and leading authorities in public health and travel medicine.

The preparation of the guidelines was coordinated by Kwon Jun Wook.

WHO gratefully acknowledges the contributions of the following:

Writing committee

Nigel Dowdall, Anthony Evans, Jose Figueroa, Kashef Ijaz, Susan Maloney, Lindsay Martinez, Corinne Ponce, Mario Raviglione, Claude Thibeault.

Review group

Léopold Blanc, Kenneth G. Castro, Dong-il Ahn, Max Hardiman, Philip Hopewell, Michael F. Iademarco, Phyllis Kozarsky, Sang-Jae Kim, Woo-jin Lew, Toru Mori, Akihiro Seita, Robert Steffen, Jeroen van Gorkom, Jane Zuckerman.

Contributors

Eric Bertherat, Neville Byrne, Keiji Fukada, Terri Hyde, Alicia Fry, Ernesto Jaramillo, William Perea, Nancy Rosenstein, Cathy Roth, Krystyna Ryszewska, Peter Strebel.

Glossary and abbreviations

acid-fast bacilli (AFB). Rod-shaped bacteria that do not lose their stain when exposed to acid or acid–alcohol mixture after the staining process, i.e. bacteria of the *Mycobacterium tuberculosis* complex and all non-tuberculous mycobacteria.

air crew. Personnel of an airline who are employed for duties on board the aircraft, including:

- **cabin crew:** personnel working in the cabin
- **flight crew:** personnel working in the cockpit

airborne. The dissemination of microbial aerosols to a suitable portal of entry, usually respiratory tract. (Droplets that settle out are not considered to be airborne.)

APU. Auxillary power unit

bacille Calmette-Guérin (BCG). A live vaccine against TB derived from an attenuated strain of *Mycobacterium bovis.*

CDC. Centers for Disease Control and Prevention, Atlanta, GA, USA

close contact. A person who has shared the same air space in an enclosed environment for a prolonged period (more than 8 hours) with a person with suspected or confirmed TB disease and who is therefore considered to be at risk of infection with *M. tuberculosis.*

contact tracing. The process of identifying close contacts of index cases, for which public health measures (such as tuberculin skin testing, chest radiography or interferon-gamma release assays) may be required.

epidemic. The occurrence in a community of a number of cases of an illness that are clearly in excess of the expected rate.

flight duration. The period commencing when an aircraft moves under its own power after leaving the stand before take-off until it is parked on the stand and the door opens after landing.

- **total flight duration:** the period including ground delays after boarding, flight duration and ground delays after landing.

haemoptysis. Coughing blood or sputum containing blood.

HEPA. High-efficiency particulate air

IATA. International Air Transport Association

ICAO. International Civil Aviation Organization

IHR. International Health Regulations

immigrant. A person from one country who has travelled to another country with the intention of settling there.

index patient. The first patient in a family or other defined group to come to the attention of the investigator.

interferon-gamma release assay. An assay for cell-mediated immunity to TB that measures interferon-gamma (IFN-γ) released from peripheral blood T-cells stimulated in vitro with TB antigens.

Mycobacterium tuberculosis. The bacterium of the *M. tuberculosis* complex that is the most common causative infectious agent of TB disease in humans. The *M. tuberculosis* complex also includes *M. bovis* and five other related species.

outbreak. The occurrence in a community or region of cases of an illness clearly in excess of normal expectation. (A localized as opposed to generalized epidemic.)

preventive therapy (for people with latent TB infection). The treatment of subclinical, latent infection with *M. tuberculosis* to prevent progression to active TB disease, usually based on 6–9 months of oral isoniazid.

SARS. Severe acute respiratory syndrome

sputum smear examination. A laboratory technique in which sputum is smeared on glass slides and stained with an acid-fast stain (e.g. carbol-fuchsin or auramine – Ziehl-Neelsen method). Slides are subsequently examined by microscopy for the presence of AFB.

tuberculin. Purified protein derivative (PPD) – a mixture of antigens from a culture filtrate extract of *M. tuberculosis* that is used for skin testing; many of its antigens are non-species specific.

tuberculin skin test (TST). Cutaneous (intradermal) injection of PPD to identify people who have been sensitized to mycobacterial antigens by infection with *M. tuberculosis*, non-tuberculous mycobacteria or vaccination with BCG.

tuberculosis (TB). The disease caused by bacteria belonging to the *M. tuberculosis* complex (*M. tuberculosis, M. bovis, M. africanum, M. microti, M. canetii, M. caprae, M. pinnipedii*), manifested by clinical, radiological or laboratory evidence with or without positive TST.

- **active TB:** tuberculosis disease associated with symptoms or signs, including findings on physical examination.
- **infectious TB:** active tuberculosis that is transmissible to others, i.e. contagious, usually determined by a positive sputum smear in case of pulmonary or laryngeal disease.
- **laryngeal TB:** tuberculosis affecting the larynx.
- **latent TB Infection:** infection with *M. tuberculosis*, diagnosed by a positive TST or serum antigen-stimulated IFN-γ release assay without clinical evidence of disease.
- **multidrug-resistant TB (MDR-TB):** tuberculosis caused by strains of *M. tuberculosis* that are resistant to at least isoniazid and rifampicin.
- **pulmonary TB:** tuberculosis involving the lung parenchyma.

universal precautions. Defined measures intended to prevent or reduce the risk of infectious exposure to blood and body fluids.

Summary

International travel has become increasingly easy and readily available. Ever greater numbers of people are using international air travel for many reasons including business, tourism, immigration, asylum seeking or humanitarian activities. There is a potential risk of transmission of tuberculosis (TB) and some other airborne or droplet-spread diseases on board commercial aircraft, particularly during long flights. Infections and in some instances outbreaks following exposure during a flight have been documented. Potential exposure to serious infectious diseases on commercial aircraft is of concern for passengers, crew and public health officials.

Reported episodes of potential transmission of TB infection during air travel in 1992–1994, and more recently the outbreak of severe acute respiratory syndrome (SARS) in 2003, raised considerable anxiety among travellers, health authorities, airline companies and the mass media. On these occasions, medical authorities, airline representatives and members of the public sought guidance from WHO and other national and international agencies. There is evidence that transmission of *Mycobacterium tuberculosis* infection may occur during long flights from an infectious source (a passenger or crew with infectious pulmonary or laryngeal TB) to other passengers or crew members. However, no case of clinical or bacteriologically confirmed TB disease has been identified as a result of air travel-related exposure during flight.

TB infection is acquired through inhalation of *M. tuberculosis* in aerosolized respiratory secretions from a contagious person coughing, talking or sneezing. The risk of infection is related to the infectiousness of the person with TB, the duration of exposure, the proximity to the source person, the ventilation and the degree of crowding. The quality of the air on board commercial aircraft is high, and under normal conditions cabin air is cleaner than the air in most buildings. On short flights, there is minimal risk of disease transmission. Prolonged journeys (i.e. more than eight hours) in a confined aircraft cabin may involve an increased risk of transmission of *M. tuberculosis*. This risk should be similar to that in other circumstances where people are together in other confined spaces.

The revised guidelines address the concerns about transmission of TB during air travel and provide the following: (i) information on transmission of TB on aircraft; (ii) a summary of the practices adopted for the management of patients with infectious TB associated with air travel, and of commonly encountered difficulties; (iii) suggestions on practical ways to reduce the risk of exposure to *M. tuberculosis* on board commercial aircraft, and (iv) guidance on procedures to follow and responsibilities when infectious TB is diagnosed in a patient who has a history of recent air travel, including contact tracing, notifying and screening for possible interventions. It also introduces the revised International Health Regulations, adopted by the World Health Assembly in May 2005, which will enter into force in June 2007, establishing basic rules for international coordination in the detection, investigation, and response to public health risks including the area of communication and information sharing.

The guidelines include specific recommendations for passengers, air crews, physicians, health authorities and airline companies. They are applicable to all domestic and international airlines worldwide.

1. Background information

Millions of people travel by air every year. It is not possible to medically assess the majority before their flights.

Approximately one third of the world's population is infected with *M. tuberculosis*, and TB is the leading cause of death from a single infectious disease agent in adults worldwide (*1*). In 2003, 4 million new and relapse TB cases were reported to WHO, of which 1.9 million were sputum smear-positive pulmonary cases. However, it is estimated that nearly 9 million cases may have occurred worldwide. More than 95% of these cases occurred in developing countries (*2*). The ease, availability and duration of air travel, with large numbers of people travelling internationally, increase the likelihood of exposure to people with infectious TB and other airborne and droplet-borne diseases.

Some industrialized countries require medical examinations for immigrants, refugees and asylum seekers, including screening for TB. Some countries also require medical examination for entering students, people on temporary work visas and visitors staying longer than three months. The timing and specific requirements of the medical examination vary from country to country. Some countries (e.g. Australia, Canada and the United States of America) require TB screening to be done in the country of origin (a chest radiograph, tuberculin test) for adolescents and adults, and sputum smear examination if the chest radiograph is suggestive of TB disease. No person with a positive smear examination is permitted to immigrate. Since these medical clearances may be valid for up to one year (e.g. for immigration to the United States), a person could develop infectious TB in the period elapsing between the medical examination and travel. Some countries (e.g. Switzerland, United Arab Emirates and the United Kingdom) screen immigrants and refugees when they enter the country; a few countries require medical examination both in the country of origin and when entering (e.g. Bahrain, Kuwait, Qatar and

Saudi Arabia). Thus, people with infectious TB would often be identified as having infectious TB only after they have travelled.

While screening for TB is usually mandatory for immigrants and refugees, the overwhelming majority of passengers flying on commercial aircraft do not fall into any category for which screening is a requirement. The International Civil Aviation Organization (ICAO) has forecast that there will be more than 2.5 billion air passengers per year by 2015 (*3*) – clearly, medical examination of the millions of people travelling by air worldwide would not be possible.

2. Tuberculosis on aircraft

Most evidence indicates that airborne transmission of infectious diseases on board aircraft appears to be limited to close personal contact and/or close proximity.

Research has shown that there is a very small risk of any infectious disease being transmitted on board aircraft (*4*). However, transmission probably occurs more frequently than reported because most diseases have an incubation period longer than the duration of air travel. Of the airborne and droplet-borne diseases that are potentially transmissible on board aircraft, the most important are TB, influenza, meningococcal disease and measles (*5*).

TB is an infectious disease, caused in most cases by *M. tuberculosis* and transmitted by exposure to tubercle bacilli in airborne droplet nuclei produced by a person with infectious TB during expiratory efforts, such as coughing, sneezing or singing. TB develops in the human body in two stages: first, the individual exposed to *M. tuberculosis* becomes infected; second, the infected individual develops the disease. However, only a small minority of infected individuals will develop the disease. While the subsequent risk of progressive TB is greatest within the first year or two after infection, latent infection may persist for life.

The latent period between acquiring TB infection and developing active TB (i.e. in the minority of infected people who go on to develop the disease) varies between 2 weeks and several decades. Primary TB occurs between 4 and 12 weeks after infection, and this can be confirmed by a demonstrable primary lesion or conversion of the tuberculin skin test. The majority of patients who ultimately develop TB will do so within the first five years after infection.

To date, no case of active TB has been identified as a result of exposure on a commercial aircraft. Furthermore, no evidence of TB disease has been reported among those known to have been infected with *M. tuberculosis* during air travel. From 1992 to 1994, the United States Centers for Disease Control and Prevention (CDC), together with state and local health departments, conducted seven contact investigations, one centred on a cabin crew member and six on passengers with infectious TB who had flown during this period. Concern was raised that the closed aircraft cabin environment may have enhanced transmission of *M. tuberculosis* (*6–11*). The number of potentially exposed passengers and cabin crew exceeded 2600 on a total of 191 flights involving nine different types of aircraft.

All index patients were highly infectious, i.e. smears from spontaneous sputum specimens from all index cases were heavily positive for acid-fast bacilli (AFB) and all patients were culture-positive and had evidence of extensive pulmonary disease on chest radiography. One patient also had biopsy- and culture-confirmed laryngeal TB, the most infectious form of TB.

In two instances, strains of *M. tuberculosis* resistant to at least isoniazid and rifampicin were isolated, i.e. multidrug-resistant tuberculosis (MDR-TB) (*7, 10*). Organisms isolated from the other patients were sensitive to all anti-TB drugs. Two passengers, who were flying to the United States for medical care, knew that they had active TB at the time of their flights but did not inform the airline of their disease. In the other five cases, TB was diagnosed after the flights.

In only two of the investigations was there evidence to suggest transmission of *M. tuberculosis* infection: one from a cabin crew member to other crew members, and another from a passenger to other passengers (*6, 10*). In the first report, evidence of transmission was limited to cabin crew with at least 12 hours' exposure to the infectious source. In the other, transmission of infection occurred to only a few passengers seated in the same section as and in close proximity to the passenger with infectious TB, and only on one flight lasting more than eight hours.

These results suggest that the risk of infection with *M. tuberculosis* during air travel is similar to that associated with other activities in which contact with potentially infectious individuals may occur (e.g. train travel, bus travel, any gathering in enclosed spaces). No case of TB disease has been reported among the infected people in the seven studies carried out by CDC. No other instances of possible TB transmission on aircraft have been published since then.

Other potentially serious airborne or droplet-transmitted infections that could merit public health interventions if encountered during air travel are influenza (both seasonal influenza and any unusual strain such as avian influenza affecting humans), measles, meningococcal disease and SARS. Box 1 presents a short description of these diseases. For further information and advice for travellers, see *International travel and health* (http://www.who.int/ith).

BOX 1

Other potentially serious airborne or droplet-spread infections

INFLUENZA is an acute viral disease of the respiratory tract spread predominantly by large respiratory droplets. Symptoms include rapid onset of fever, headache, myalgia (muscle pain), sore throat, cough and often coryza (nasal mucus). Air travel can be a vehicle for the global spread of influenza strains and transmission can take place aboard aircraft. An outbreak occurred in 1979 among passengers on a flight that was delayed for three hours on the ground before take-off (*12*). The attack rate among passengers was high (72%) and was associated with the ventilation system not being in operation during the ground delay. Since December 2003, cases of highly pathogenic avian influenza affecting humans (mostly influenza A, H5N1) have been reported in countries in Asia, Europe and the Middle East. No sustained person-to-person transmission of avian influenza has been identified.

MEASLES is an acute, highly infectious airborne viral disease. It has an incubation period of 10–12 days (range 7–18 days) from exposure to onset of symptoms and a prodromal phase of 2–4 days with nonspecific symptoms such as fever and malaise. The characteristic rash appears on the body between the third and seventh day of symptoms. Measles can be transmitted from 4 days before to 4 days after appearance of the rash; transmission is minimal after the second day of rash. Non-immunized people, especially young children, are at highest risk for measles and its complications, including death.

MENINGOCOCCAL DISEASE (including meningococcal meningitis and septicaemia) is an acute bacterial disease caused by *Neisseria meningitidis* transmitted from person to person through droplets, either by inhalation or by direct contact with respiratory secretions (e.g. during mouth-to-mouth resuscitation) or infected blood. Early signs and symptoms are nonspecific and difficult to differentiate from influenza or other common diseases. The incubation period varies from 2–10 days (usually 3–5 days). Cases of air travel-related meningococcal disease have been reported (*13*).

SARS is a recently recognized severe acute pneumonia caused by a SARS-associated coronavirus; it manifested as a single epidemic affecting 8000 people in 29 countries in 2002–2003, constituting a major international public health emergency. The epidemic originated in southern China, and the virus is considered to have an unconfirmed animal reservoir. The epidemic was spread globally by air travellers and possible cases of in-flight transmission were reported (*14*). SARS is believed to have been spread by droplets either by close person-to-person contact or indirectly by contact with fomites (objects or materials that are likely to carry infection), although airborne or small droplet transmission could not be excluded. Symptoms developed within 10 days of exposure. Initial symptoms were systemic (fever, malaise, myalgia, diarrhoea); respiratory symptoms developed a few days later. Patients are thought to have been most infectious during the second week of illness.

3. Practical issues in conducting investigations concerning exposure to *M. tuberculosis*

Adequate and timely contact tracing after potential exposure to *M. tuberculosis* may be impeded by practical constraints, particularly the length of time between travel and diagnosis and the accuracy and availability of airline records.

Investigations of possible *M. tuberculosis* transmission aboard commercial aircraft are usually initiated several weeks to months after the flight. Passengers are therefore often difficult to locate. With the exception of passengers enrolled in "frequent flyer" programmes, airline companies do not maintain records of passengers' addresses, telephone numbers or emergency contact information. Although a telephone number is usually requested at booking, this is not an absolute requirement and the accuracy of the information provided is not known. In general, contact information maintained in airline records is inadequate in a high proportion of cases. On domestic flights it may be possible for passengers to fly under assumed names or give their tickets to other people. This is less likely to happen on international flights. The International Air Transport Association (IATA) and its partners, including WHO, are actively looking at ways to improve the accuracy and availability of passenger information.

Immigration (landing) cards are completed by passengers and crew arriving in some countries and residence addresses are required. Depending on the country, one form may be completed for passengers from the same household rather than separate forms for each individual passenger. In addition, because forms are handwritten, it is often not possible to read the passenger's name and the address information is often incomplete or missing. Thus, the usefulness of these forms for follow-up purposes is extremely limited, and contact tracing often cannot be accomplished. Efforts are under way nationally and internationally to rectify this situation. As an interim measure, locator cards are being developed: these will contain the name, seat number and emergency contact information of each passenger on board in the event that someone on the same flight may have a transmissible infectious disease of public health significance.

Substantial delays may occur between diagnosis of TB disease and recognition that a person with infectious TB disease had travelled on a commercial flight(s). Informing passengers and crew of a potential exposure to TB should be limited to flights that have occurred within the three months before notification of the TB case to the health authorities.

In situations where suspected infectious TB cases are identified on airline flights, passengers and cabin crew should be informed as soon as possible of their potential exposure to *M. tuberculosis* and encouraged to seek further medical advice.

4. Legal and regulatory issues

Airline companies are expected to comply with the International Health Regulations and the laws of the countries in which they operate.

Airline companies are expected to comply with the International Health Regulations (IHR), which are designed to prevent the international spread of disease while interfering as little as possible with travel and trade. The Regulations, revised in 2005, include several provisions that may apply to the detection and control of TB and other airborne diseases on board aircraft, as outlined in Box 2.

Airlines are also expected to comply with the laws of the countries in which they operate. It is the responsibility of airlines to be familiar with the specific laws and regulations concerning infectious diseases applying to passengers and goods at points of entry for each destination country. Similarly, when transporting infectious agents or people with infectious diseases, airline companies should comply with the laws on safety procedures and on release of passenger information of each country to which they fly.

Confidentiality must be ensured when health authorities need to release the name of a passenger with TB to an airline in order to confirm that the passenger was on a particular flight(s). This information should be communicated securely and confidentially to the airline's medical service or its designated contact person.

Confidentiality is also a concern for airline companies when health authorities request the release of passenger and crew lists. Airlines should cooperate with public health authorities, in compliance with the IHR and the laws of the countries in which they land. It is the responsibility of the public health authorities to carry out patient notification and contact tracing. They are competent to do so and are supported by the law if any enforcement is required. Furthermore, this will not break confidentiality, since a compelling public health demand overrides any individual confidentiality issue.

BOX 2

International Health Regulations, 2005

PROVISIONS RELEVANT TO TRANSMISSION OF TUBERCULOSIS ON AIRCRAFT

Preventing the international spread of disease requires early detection of unusual disease events through an effective national surveillance system as well as appropriate preparedness to respond to these events, including at international points of entry and exit.

The International Health Regulations 2005 (IHR 2005)[1] adopted by the World Health Assembly in May 2005 will enter into force in June 2007. They operate through (i) routine measures to address the continuous risks of disease spread and (ii) special measures recommended for application during a sudden heightening of specific risks, i.e. during a public health emergency of international concern.

The IHR 2005 establish basic rules for international coordination in the detection, investigation and response to public health risks, including in the area of communication and information sharing.

GENERAL PROVISIONS RELEVANT TO TB AND AIR TRAVEL

The scope of the IHR 2005 (Article 2) includes acute public health emergencies and public health risks that present a serious and direct danger to human health and that may spread internationally. TB and other airborne diseases can fall within the scope of the IHR 2005, and a number of provisions are of relevance to measures for their detection and control during international travel.

Diseases transmitted primarily by the airborne route are of concern when groups of people are kept in confined spaces for prolonged periods of time, such as during long-distance air travel. The key IHR 2005 provisions pertinent to these diseases and air travel are summarized below.

- **Information-sharing requirements**

States Parties may require, for public health purposes, on arrival or on departure:

— travellers to provide information on their itinerary and destination (Article 23);

— conveyances and conveyance operators to share relevant public health information. Such information may include passenger manifests and seating plans, which may be needed for contact tracing and follow-up after an infectious person has travelled by air (Annex1).

Officers in command of aircraft are obliged to report any cases of illness indicative of a public health risk on board as early as possible before arrival at the airport of destination. This information must be relayed immediately to the competent authorities for the airport (Article 28.4). Conveyance operators shall use the Health Part of the Aircraft General Declaration to inform airport authorities when so requested or as appropriate.

[1] http://www.who.int/csr/ihr/en/

- **Notification of disease**

It is noted here that States Parties are required to notify WHO of any potential public health emergency of international concern as defined in Annex 2 of the IHR 2005. Of the airborne diseases, Annex 2 lists SARS as a disease that, at this time, would always be considered as a potential public health emergency of international concern and require notification. Meningococcal disease is included in a separate list of disease entities, the occurrence of which must always prompt States to undertake an assessment, using the above-mentioned decision instrument, of the need to notify WHO under the Regulations. TB is not listed in Annex 2, but the assessment would be applied in the event of a potential international emergency due to TB.

- **Treatment of personal data**

States Parties are obliged to collect and handle health information containing personal identifiers in a confidential manner. However, States Parties may disclose and process personal data where it is essential for the purposes of assessing and managing a public health risk (Article 45).

HEALTH MEASURES APPLIED TO TRAVELLERS

- **Medical examination**

States Parties may require, for public health purposes, travellers on arrival or on departure to undergo a medical examination to determine whether or not they constitute a public health risk (Article 23). This would include a sputum test, when justified.

- **Suspected or affected travellers**

A State Party may apply additional health measures on the basis of evidence of a public health risk, in particular with regard to suspect or affected travellers (Article 23). In the context of the IHR 2005, an "affected traveller" is a traveller who is infected or contaminated or who carries sources of infection or contamination, so as to constitute a public health risk. A "suspected traveller" is a traveller who has been exposed, or possibly exposed, to a public health risk and who could be a possible source of spread of disease (Article 1).

- **Travellers seeking temporary or permanent residence**

These Regulations do not preclude States Parties from requiring additional medical examination, vaccination or other prophylaxis or proof of vaccination as a condition of entry for any traveller seeking temporary or permanent residence.

- **Informed consent**

In all cases, no medical examination or other health measures shall be carried out without a traveller's prior express informed consent (Article 23). However, if the traveller fails to consent to any measures or refuses to provide the information or documents needed, the State Party may deny entry to the traveller (Article 31). If there is evidence that the traveller poses an imminent public health risk, a State Party may compel the traveller to undergo a medical examination, vaccination or other prophylaxis or additional health measures (Article 31).

- **Treatment of travellers**

States Parties shall treat travellers with respect for their dignity, human rights and fundamental freedoms and minimize any discomfort or distress associated with such measures (Article 32).

- **Charges for health measures regarding travellers**

With the exception of those seeking temporary or permanent residence, the IHR 2005 prohibit the levying of charges for certain prescribed measures applied for the protection of the public's health. However, States Parties may charge for other health measures including those that are primarily for the benefit of the traveller according to certain rules established in the Regulations (Article 40).

WHO RECOMMENDATIONS UNDER THE IHR 2005

WHO may make recommendations under the IHR 2005 (Articles 16–18) for the application of measures by States Parties or by operators of international transport. The IHR 2005 define two types of recommendations depending on the nature of the public health risk:

— Temporary recommendations are made by WHO on an ad hoc, time-limited, risk basis, in response to a public health emergency of international concern.

— Standing recommendations indicate the appropriate measures for specific ongoing public health risks for routine or periodic application, including at international points of entry.

WHO may issue recommendations under the IHR 2005 detailing specific measures for application in respect of air travel and the transmission of the diseases included in this guideline either in response to a sudden event (temporary recommendations) or for routine application (standing recommendations).

Although the captain of an aircraft can legally deny boarding to a person if he or she has a valid concern that the person is a threat to the health and/or safety of other passengers and crew, in practice this may be difficult to apply. If a passenger is obviously very ill and with signs and/or symptoms suggesting an infectious disease, a medical consultation may be obtained before boarding. National laws vary significantly in different countries and air crew may be hesitant to deny boarding when privacy concerns may protect the individual passenger and discrimination charges may be an issue. However, many countries have laws or regulations to prevent people known to have infectious TB from boarding commercial aircraft.

Boarding can and should be denied to individuals with an infectious form of TB. When a physician is aware that a person with an infectious form of TB is planning to travel on a commercial carrier, he or she should inform the public health authority who in turn should inform the airline concerned. To avoid false reports of a malicious nature, airlines should require a written notification from the public health authorities.

5. Reducing the risk of exposure to *M. tuberculosis* on aircraft

People known to have infectious TB must not travel by public air transportation until at least two weeks of adequate treatment have been completed. Patients with MDR-TB should not travel until they have been proved to be non-infectious (i.e. culture-negative).

People known to have infectious TB should comply with the measures and policies recommended by the national TB control programme, until there is no longer a risk of transmitting infection to others. When travel is necessary while a person is still infectious, commercial carriers or other public transportation should not be used. Alternative private transportation (e.g. ground transportation, air ambulance, private carrier) could be used instead. If the use of commercial aviation is unavoidable, a specific protocol should be established by the national public health authorities in cooperation with the airline.

People with TB are often infectious long before the disease is diagnosed. Aircraft passengers with undiagnosed TB will therefore not be identified as infectious before boarding. Symptoms of TB disease (e.g. cough) are not specific. Even if airline staff asked all passengers and crew about such symptoms, it is not possible or appropriate for them to decide whether or not a person has infectious TB. Unless the passenger is obviously ill, it would be difficult to determine whether he or she is medically unfit to travel. Thus, passengers with infectious TB are more likely to be identified after, rather than at the time of, a flight.

Denying boarding to all TB patients under treatment would not be justified. The majority of TB cases become non-infectious after two weeks of adequate treatment (*16*, *17*). Although patients infected with MDR-TB will require a longer period of adequate treatment and detailed follow-up, denying boarding to a patient under treatment for MDR-TB is not justified provided the patient is culture-negative, which indicates reduced risk of transmission.

Physicians should inform all infectious TB patients that they must not travel by air until they have completed at least two weeks of adequate treatment. Patients with MDR-TB should be advised not to travel until proven by adequate laboratory confirmation (i.e. culture) to be non-infectious.

Transmission of TB has been documented only in flights lasting longer than eight hours. If travel on a short flight during the first two weeks of treatment is essential (e.g. going to a tertiary care facility for further investigation or returning home to an isolated area when asymptomatic), a protocol should be agreed between the airline involved and the public health authorities.

If during a flight a passenger is suspected of having infectious TB because he or she informs the cabin crew of, or experiences, severe symptoms such as haemoptysis, the cabin crew should try to relocate the passenger in a more comfortable and isolated area if space is available. One cabin crew member should be designated to look after the ill passenger, preferably the crew member who has already been dealing with him or her. The ill passenger should be given a surgical face mask. If no mask is available or if the mask cannot be tolerated, the passenger should be given an adequate supply of paper handkerchiefs (or towels if necessary) and instructed to cover his or her nose and mouth at least when speaking or coughing. The cabin crew should follow standard universal precautions when handling potentially infectious material (e.g. wear gloves, place disposables in sealed plastic bags) (*18*). The designated cabin crew member may wear a mask if available, especially if the ill person cannot tolerate a mask. The IATA guidelines for suspected communicable disease in-flight, which have been approved by WHO, should always be followed by all airlines (*19*).

6. Aircraft ventilation

In case of ground delays of more than 30 minutes, adequate cabin ventilation must be ensured.

While an aircraft is parked at the stand with the engines off, passenger cabin ventilation is normally supplied by one of the following means: (i) an air conditioning unit (preconditioned air source) connected to the aircraft ventilation system; (ii) a ground pneumatic source providing the air required to operate the aircraft environmental control system; (iii) the auxiliary power unit (APU) of the aircraft running the aircraft ventilation system; (iv) natural airflow through the aircraft's open door(s), usually for short periods and only when no other source of ventilation is available.

Once the aircraft has left the stand and the engines have been started, the APU is shut down and the air supply to the cabin is drawn from some compressor stages of the engines. This "bleed" air supply is at high pressure and temperature (ranging from 150 °C to 280 °C, depending on the stage of flight) and the environmental system cools and conditions the air to comfortable levels before introducing it into the passenger cabin. Air is distributed evenly throughout the passenger cabin via ducts running the entire length of the aircraft. Air enters the cabin from overhead distribution outlets and flows downwards in a circular pattern towards the outflow grills along both sidewalls of the cabin near the floor (Figure 1). Air enters and leaves the cabin at approximately the same seat row, and airflow in fore and aft directions is minimal. Movement of passengers and crew in the cabin has minimal impact on the intended airflow patterns.

When the aircraft is delayed on the ground and the doors are closed, the ventilation system should be operating. An influenza outbreak on an aircraft was greatly facilitated by a ground delay lasting three hours, during which the ventilation system did not operate and the passengers did not receive outside air (*12*). Thus, ground delays without adequate ventilation must be kept as short as possible. According to a study by the United States Department of Transportation: "If the ventilation system is not operating, passengers should not stay aboard the plane for long time periods (i.e. greater than 30 minutes)" (*20*).

All commercial jet aircraft built after the late 1980s, and a few adapted older aircraft, recirculate the cabin air: from 10% to 50% of the cabin air is filtered, mixed with outside conditioned bleed air from the engine compressors and then reintroduced into the passenger cabin. Depending on the type of aircraft, air may be recirculated throughout the entire cabin or only within limited zones. All large commercial jet aircraft provide approximately 20 air exchanges per hour during cruising, with lower amounts during descent and on the ground.

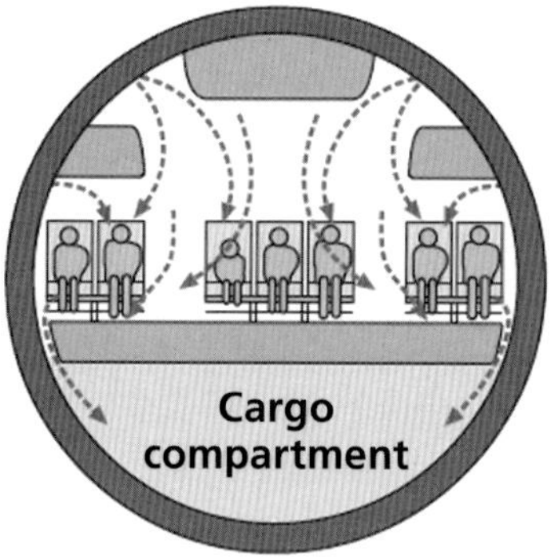

Figure 1. Cabin airflow patterns

7. Cabin air quality

There is no evidence that recirculation of cabin air facilitates transmission of infectious disease agents on board.

Airline crew, passengers and the media have expressed concern about possible health risks to passengers and crew relating to air contaminants and air recirculation on aircraft. At cruising altitude, outside ambient air is virtually free of microorganisms. When recirculated, the cabin air passes through a set of filters before being mixed with outside conditioned air and re-entering the passenger cabin. Generally, the first filter (or pre-filter) traps the largest particles. Subsequently, on most modern aircraft, the air passes through high-efficiency particulate air (HEPA) filters before re-entering the passenger cabin. The most efficient HEPA filters will capture 99.99% of particles (bacteria, fungi, and larger viruses) between 0.1 and 0.3 µm. The tubercle bacillus is approximately 0.5–1 µm in size. Therefore, HEPA filters remove any *M. tuberculosis* organisms from the re-circulating air, thus eliminating the risk of exposure for passengers and crew from this source.

A few studies have examined microbial contaminants in aircraft cabin air. No evidence has been found that microbial contamination of cabin air entails a greater risk of disease transmission aboard a commercial aircraft than in any other public setting (*20–22*). The concentrations of bacteria and fungi found are so low that they are not thought to pose any health risk: they are sometimes lower than those found in other public places or in private houses. This has been attributed to the sterility of the air entering the aircraft at cruising altitude, to the high airflow rates and the laminar (non-turbulent) airflow pattern in the passenger cabin and to the high-efficiency filters used for recirculated air.

Passengers on the aircraft are the most important source of any microbial aerosols in the cabin air. Droplet nuclei containing *M. tuberculosis* bacteria are aerosolized in the cabin air when a person with infectious TB coughs or speaks. Droplet nuclei will then follow the airflow in the passenger cabin. If there is no airflow, microorganisms can remain dispersed in the air for some time (*12*). In most modern aircraft, however, when the ventilation system is operating, air is recirculated and filtered at high rate, and any airborne particles would be rapidly removed. It has been shown that after a sudden increase in bacterial concentration (e.g. after a cough or a sneeze), all measurements return to normal levels within three minutes (*21*).

Investigations of possible transmission of *M. tuberculosis* on aircraft (*6–10*) found no evidence that it was facilitated by recirculation of the cabin air. In the only report of probable passenger-to-passenger transmission, *M. tuberculosis* infection was identified for only a few passengers seated in the same section of the aircraft as the infected passenger. The aircraft used on this flight recirculated up to 50% of the air in the passenger cabin throughout the entire aircraft, and air from the rear section was recirculated in the front section. In reported investigations of measles transmission on aircraft, only passengers seated within a few rows of the ill passenger were infected (*23, 24*). However, a report on SARS transmission on aircraft (*14*) showed that cases occurred among passengers seated further apart and on flights lasting considerably less than 8 hours. The possibility that passengers who developed SARS were infected before or after the flight could not be excluded.

8. Procedures for informing passengers and crew when exposure to *M. tuberculosis* is suspected

It is recommended that airline companies cooperate with public health authorities that are responsible for informing passengers and/or crew of their potential exposure to *M. tuberculosis*.

Health authorities and the airline medical service (or designated official) should work together to determine whether an exposure to TB could have occurred and, if so, which passengers or crew members should be informed. In all situations, health authorities should make the final decision. Airlines should collaborate closely with health authorities in ensuring that all possible contacts receive appropriate information promptly.

The following guidelines are designed to assist health authorities in determining when passengers and crew should be informed of their possible exposure to infectious TB on commercial flights (Figure 2).

8.1 Communication between health authorities and airlines

Health authorities are usually the first to receive information about a person (cabin crew or passenger) in whom TB has been diagnosed. However, if the airline is informed first, it should advise the informant (patient, physician, others) that the treating physician must communicate all information immediately to the health authorities. Before any further action is considered in such cases, health authorities must confirm whether the person has pulmonary or laryngeal TB likely to have been infectious at the time of the flight. After confirmation of the case, the health authority should communicate with the counterpart authorities in all countries where there may have been a risk of exposure. Contact tracing and careful follow-up are particularly important in the case of infectious MDR-TB as case management is more complex and challenging.

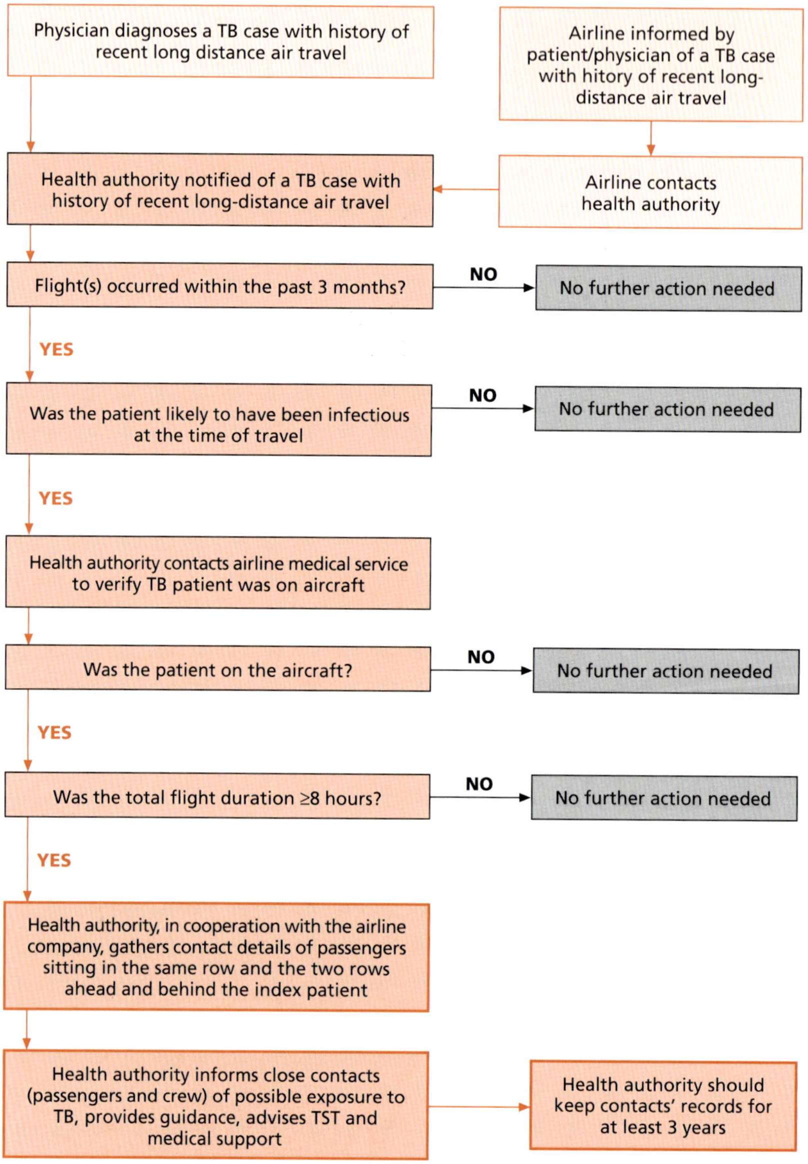

Figure 2. Steps to follow when deciding whether contact tracing is needed

8.2 Criteria for deciding whether to inform passengers and crew

Once notified, the health authorities must evaluate the risk of *M. tuberculosis* transmission and decide whether it is necessary to inform passengers and crew of the potential exposure. For this purpose, the following criteria should be used:

- infectiousness of the person with TB;
- duration of exposure;
- time elapsed between the flight(s) and the notification of the case;
- proximity of other passengers and crew to the index patient.

8.2.1 Infectiousness of the person with TB

Determination of infectiousness. Tracing passengers and crew and informing them of potential exposure to *M. tuberculosis* are recommended only if the person with TB is likely to have been infectious at the time of the flight(s). The infectiousness of the index case is to be assessed by the relevant health authorities. A person should be considered infectious at the time of the flight(s) when he or she meets the conditions identified in the following algorithm (Table 1).

8.2.2 Duration of exposure

Informing close contacts is indicated if total flight duration exceeded 8 hours. After the health authorities have concluded that the person could have been infectious at the time of the flight(s), they should contact the airline medical consultant (or other designated staff) promptly in order to confirm that the person with TB was on the flight(s) in question and to determine the total duration of the flight(s).

When estimating the duration of exposure, the total duration of the flight, including ground delays after boarding, flying time and ground delays after landing, must be taken into account. Evidence for *M. tuberculosis* transmission has been found only when exposure to the person with TB exceeded eight hours (*10*). Therefore, health authorities and airline medical consultants may consider informing only passengers and crew exposed for at least eight hours. If the TB patient travelled on more than one airline and each flight time was more than eight hours, the public health authority should contact each airline.

If the total flight time exceeded eight hours, the public health authority should send an official letter to the airline company requesting passenger contact information. A sample letter is provided in Annex 1.

8.2.3 Time elapsed between the flight(s) and the notification of the case

Informing passengers and crew should be limited to flights that took place during the three months before notification of the TB case to the health authorities. Determining retrospectively whether a person with TB was symptomatic at the time of the flight(s) can be very difficult, and the reliability of the information will be related to the time interval between the flight and the diagnosis of TB. There may be substantial delays between diagnosis of TB and recognition that the person with infectious TB had travelled on a commercial flight(s).

In the assessment of a positive TST result, other possible reasons must be considered besides recent infection with *M. tuberculosis*, including prior exposure to TB, residence or birth in countries in which TB is endemic, and BCG vaccination. In the United States, an estimated 4–6% of the total population is TST-positive. In developing countries, the estimated prevalence of *M. tuberculosis* infection among the general population ranges from 19% (in the WHO Eastern Mediterranean Region) to 44% (in the WHO Western Pacific Region) (*2*). A single, positive TST result does not therefore reliably represent recent infection in passengers from countries where TB is common, and further follow-up may be indicated.

Recently developed serological assays that measure interferon-gamma (IFN-γ) release could be used for screening for latent TB infection in countries of low endemicity (*25, 26*). These assays are based on the fact that T-cells from the blood of people who have been previously sensitized to *M. tuberculosis* antigens will produce high levels of IFN-γ when re-exposed to the same antigens in vitro. New generations of these tests use *M. tuberculosis*-specific antigens that are not found in BCG or in most other non-tuberculous mycobacterial species.

Given the difficulties in (i) assessing infectiousness at the time of the flight, (ii) interpreting TST results, and (iii) obtaining sufficiently accurate passenger travel and seating details, three months is considered the maximum time after travel that would warrant public health intervention, including contacting the airlines and subsequent contact tracing.

Table 1. Laboratory and clinical conditions under which TB patients should be considered infectious at the time of the flight(s)

Laboratory	Positive AFB smears from sputum specimens AND/OR Positive cultures for *M. tuberculosis* ***AND at the time of the flight***
Clinical	• Clinical symptoms of TB including cough AND • Not receiving adequate TB treatment OR • Receiving adequate TB treatment for less than 2 weeks OR • Receiving adequate TB treatment for more than 2 weeks but with no evidence of response (e.g. no clinical improvement or no documentation of sputum conversion from AFB smear-positive to AFB smear-negative). If MDR-TB • Not receiving adequate treatment OR • Receiving adequate treatment for any length of time but with no evidence of culture conversion.

8.2.4 Proximity of other passengers and crew to the index patient

Passenger-to-passenger transmission of *M. tuberculosis* has been documented only among close contacts seated in the same section as the person with infectious TB. Informing those passengers seated in the same row as the index patient and those seated in the two rows ahead and behind, as well as cabin crew members working in the same cabin section, will therefore usually be sufficient. However, in some instances a larger number of passengers and crew may need to be informed, depending on the total duration of the flight, including any ground delays, the activities of the infectious TB person aboard and the specific seating configuration of the aircraft involved.

Passengers are not considered to be close contacts if the infectious source is one of the flight crew (i.e. pilot, co-pilot, flight engineers) because there is usually no contact between passengers and flight crew. However, in such cases other crew members should be informed.

8.3 Informing passengers and crew

Public health authorities are responsible for tracing and informing close contacts (passengers or crew) of their potential exposure to *M. tuberculosis*. Airline companies should cooperate with the relevant health authorities to provide the information needed to contact all people who are likely to have been exposed so that the health authorities can provide them with appropriate information and guidance. Airlines usually have a system in place to reach passengers and inform them of flight changes or cancellations.

In all cases of severe infectious disease, the treating physician should undertake a clinical evaluation that includes a detailed travel history (including travel by air, destination(s) and duration of travel). After assessing a recent (i.e. within three months) history of air travel in a patient with confirmed TB disease, physicians should immediately inform the health authority, in addition to submitting the required notification for a TB case. Figure 2 shows a flowchart summarizing the recommended procedures for deciding whether tracing and informing passengers and crew is needed.

9. Airline employee health

The risk of TB among cabin crew members is similar to that of the general population. Mandatory routine or periodic screening is not indicated for cabin crew.

Available data about transmission of *M. tuberculosis* on aircraft do not suggest an increased risk for cabin crew resulting from their work, and thus routine and periodic tuberculin screening of all flight crew is not indicated.

When the infectious source is a crew member (i.e. cabin or flight crew), an assessment of individual work assignments should be made. All other crew with a cumulative exposure of at least eight hours during the period when the crew member with TB was potentially infectious should be informed of their exposure and advised to seek medical evaluation. Crew members would be considered close contacts if they are exposed to the infectious source while working, travelling and socializing together.

All crew should receive training about potential exposure to infectious diseases during flights and while in a foreign country. Cabin crew should also be trained in first aid and in the use of universal precautions when there may be exposure to body fluids (*18*), according to ICAO regulations. Airlines should ensure that gloves, surgical masks and biohazard disposal bags are always readily available on all aircraft. Airline cleaning staff should be prepared for appropriate cleaning of the aircraft after potentially infectious passengers have disembarked.

10. Recommendations

For passengers and air crew

1. People with infectious TB must postpone long-distance travel (total flight exceeding eight hours) until they become non-infectious (completion of at least two weeks of adequate treatment) and according to the recommendations of their physicians.
2. People with MDR-TB must postpone any air travel until advised by their physicians that they are no longer infectious, i.e. culture-negative.

For physicians

3. Physicians should inform all infectious TB patients that they must not travel by air on a flight exceeding eight hours until they have completed at least two weeks of adequate treatment.
4. Physicians should inform all MDR-TB patients that they must not travel by air – under any circumstances or on a flight of any duration – until they are proven to be culture-negative.
5. Physicians should advise TB patients who undertake unavoidable air travel of short duration (less than eight hours) to wear a surgical mask when possible or to cover the nose and mouth when speaking or coughing at all times during the flight.
6. Physicians should inform the relevant health authority when they are aware of an infectious TB patient's intention to travel against medical advice.
7. Physicians should immediately inform the relevant health authority when an infectious TB patient has a recent history of air travel (i.e. within three months).

For public health authorities

8. Public health authorities who are aware that a person with infectious TB is planning to travel with a commercial carrier on a flight whose total duration could potentially exceed eight hours should inform the concerned airline.

9. Health authorities should promptly contact the airline when an infectious TB patient is known to have travelled on a commercial flight of at least eight hours' duration (including ground delay time) within the preceding three months.
10. Health authorities should promptly contact potentially exposed passengers and crew and advise them to seek medical evaluation.
11. Public health authorities should establish country-specific policies and provide guidance to airlines on the prevention of risks due to infectious diseases.

For airline companies

12. Airline companies should deny boarding to any person who is known to have infectious TB and is intending to travel on a flight whose total duration is likely to be at least eight hours.
13. Airline companies should minimize ground delays to less than 30 minutes if the ventilation system is not in operation.
14. Airline companies should ensure that HEPA filters on all aircraft are changed regularly according to the recommendations of the filter manufacturer.
15. Airline companies should ensure that cabin crews receive adequate training on potential exposure to infectious diseases, in first aid and in using universal precautions when there may be exposure to body fluids.
16. Airline companies should ensure that there are adequate emergency medical supplies aboard all aircraft (including gloves, surgical masks and biohazard disposal bags).
17. Airline companies should cooperate with health authorities in providing all contact information needed by them and facilitate contact tracing of passengers and/or crew.

11. References

1. Raviglione MC, Snider DE, Kochi A. Global epidemiology of tuberculosis: morbidity and mortality of a worldwide epidemic. *Journal of the American Medical Association*, 1995, 273:220–226.
2. *Global tuberculosis control: surveillance, planning, financing*. WHO report 2005. Geneva, World Health Organization, 2005 (WHO/HTM/TB/2005.349).
3. *Outlook for air transport to the year 2015*. Montreal, International Civil Aviation Organization, 2004 (Circular 304 AT/127, 2004).
4. Mangili A, Gendreau MA. Transmission of infectious diseases during commercial air travel. *Lancet*, 2005, 365:989–996.
5. *International travel and health 2005*. Geneva, World Health Organization, 2005 (http://www.who.int/ith).
6. Driver CR et al. Transmission of M. tuberculosis associated with air travel. *Journal of the American Medical Association*, 1994, 272: 1031–1035.
7. McFarland JW et al. Exposure to *Mycobacterium tuberculosis* during air travel. *Lancet*, 1993, 342:112–113.
8. Exposure of passengers and flight crew to *Mycobacterium tuberculosis* on commercial aircraft, 1992–1995. *Morbidity and Mortality Weekly Report*, 1995, 44:137–140.
9. Miller MA, Valway SE, Onorato IM. Tuberculosis risk after exposure on airplanes. *Tubercle and Lung Disease*, 1996, 77:414–419.
10. Kenyon TA et al. Transmission of multidrug-resistant *Mycobacterium tuberculosis* during a long airplane flight. *New England Journal of Medicine*, 1996, 334:933–938.
11. Moore M, Fleming KS, Sands L. A passenger with pulmonary/laryngeal tuberculosis: no evidence of transmission on two short flights. *Aviation, Space, and Environmental Medicine*, 1996, 67:1097–1100.
12. Moser MR et al. An outbreak of influenza aboard a commercial airliner. *American Journal of Epidemiology*, 1979,110:1–6.
13. Stone SC, Kassinove AS. Exposure to patients with meningococcal disease on aircraft, United States, 1999–2001. *Annals of Emergency Medicine*, 2001, 38(5):598–599.

14. Olsen SJ et al. Transmission of severe acute respiratory syndrome on aircraft. *New England Journal of Medicine*, 2003, 349:2416–2422.
15. Rouillon A, Perdrizet S, Parot R. Transmission of tubercle bacilli: the effect of chemotherapy. *Tubercle*, 1976, 57:275–299.
16. *Treatment of tuberculosis: guidelines for national programmes*. Geneva, World Health Organization, 2003 (WHO/CDS/TB/2003.313).
17. *Guidelines for the programmatic management of drug-resistant tuberculosis*. Geneva, World Health Organization, 2006 (WHO/HTM/TB/2006.361).
18. Update: universal precautions for prevention of transmission of human immunodeficiency virus, hepatitis B virus, and other blood-borne pathogens in health care settings. *Morbidity and Mortality Weekly Report*, 1998, 37:377–388.
19. *Suspected communicable disease: general guideline for cabin crew*. Montreal, International Air Transport Association, 2005.
20. Nagda NL et al. *Airliner cabin environment: contaminant measurements, health risks and mitigation options*. Washington, DC, United States Department of Transportation, 1989 (Report number DOT-P-15-89-5).
21. Dechow M, Sohn H, Steinhauses J. Concentrations of selected contaminants in cabin air of Airbus aircraft. *Chemosphere*, 1997, 35: 21–31.
22. Wick RL Jr, Irvine LA. The microbiological composition of airliner cabin air. *Aviation, Space, and Environmental Medicine*, 1995, 66:220–224.
23. Amler RW et al. Imported measles in the United States. *Journal of the American Medical Association*, 1982, 248:2219–2233.
24. Interstate importation of measles following transmission in an airport – California, Washington, 1982. *Morbidity and Mortality Weekly Report*, 1983, 32(16):215–216.
25. Pai M, Riley LW, Colford JM Jr. Interferon-gamma assays in the immunodiagnosis of tuberculosis: a systematic review. *Lancet Infectious Diseases*, 2004, 4(12):761–776.
26. Guidelines for using the QuantiFERON®-TB Gold Test for detecting *Mycobacterium tuberculosis* infection, United States. *Morbidity and Mortality Weekly Report*, 2005, 54(RR15):49–55.

Annex I

Sample letter from a health authority to an airline company requesting information for contact tracing after possible exposure to *M. tuberculosis*

N.B. This official letter should normally be sent only after the health authority has confirmed with the airline company that a TB patient likely to have been infectious was on board within the past three months and that the flight lasted more than eight hours.

Date ....

Address of airline medical consultant

Dear colleague,

We have recently been notified of a case of tuberculosis (TB) with a recent history of air travel. This patient has been judged to have been infectious at the time of the flight.

The patient, **[Mr/Ms ....]**, reported flying from **[town/airport of departure]** to **[town/airport of landing]** on **[date]** on your flight **[flight details – flight number and/or seat number if available – as precise as possible]**.

It was also confirmed that the flight in question was of more than **eight hours**' total duration. There is some evidence that transmission of *Mycobacterium tuberculosis* may occur during long (more than eight hours) flights, from an infectious source (passenger or crew member) to other passengers and crew members.

Thus, **all cabin crew** who were on this flight and in the same cabin section as the patient and at least **all passengers seated in the same row and those seated in the two rows in front of and two rows behind the index patient** are to be considered *flight* contacts and potentially exposed to TB.

Would you kindly provide us with the contact information for all of these individuals (names, addresses of origin and destination, telephone numbers). The information will be used on a strictly confidential basis to provide medical guidance to those concerned.

Thank you for your cooperation.

Yours sincerely,

[Name, address, telephone/fax number of health authority]